THE DREADED WOMEN INFECTIONS:
7 Most Prevalent Kinds Of Infections, Symptoms, Causes And Prevention.

Dr. John E. Fuller

Table of contents

CHAPTER ONE

VAGINAL INFLAMMATION "VAGINITIS"

It's usual for women to encounter vaginal difficulties on an infrequent basis. Vaginal difficulties may emerge from fluctuations in menstrual cycles, from intercourse with a new partner, and even from birth control. The vagina is a sensitive, self-cleansing component of female sexual organs but every so often, a woman may realize her vagina is not operating the way it generally does.

She may notice discharge, a strange scent, or a feeling that includes burning, itching, or other discomforts. Sometimes a lady is unaware whether vaginal sexually transmitted illnesses have harmed her well-being and sometimes, she may be concerned and the question "Are yeast infections contagious?"

Various common infections may lead to vaginal illnesses, therefore you must contact women's health specialists, who are not only well-versed in gynecological therapy but also treat women holistically, considering the many causes that might set off vaginal troubles.

What Are Common Types of Vaginal Issues?

Many forms of vaginal disorders may emerge during a woman's life. Some vaginal disorders, such vaginal sexually transmitted diseases, might be more severe in terms of symptoms than other vaginal issues, like yeast infections. You may question – are yeast infections contagious.

VAGINITIS

Vaginitis is a name for numerous conditions that cause inflammation or infection of your vagina. These may be produced by organisms like yeast or bacteria, or by irritations from chemicals or sprays.

What Is Vaginitis?

Vaginitis is a medical word that covers several illnesses that cause your vagina to become infected or inflamed. Vulvovaginitis refers to inflammation of both the vagina and vulva (the exterior female genitals) (the external female genitals). These diseases may occur from an infection produced by organisms like bacteria, yeast, or viruses. Irritations from chemicals in lotions, sprays, or even garments that come in touch with this region may also result in vaginitis. In certain circumstances, vaginitis develops from organisms that are transferred between sexual partners, vaginal dryness, and lack of estrogen.

The most prevalent kinds of vaginitis are:
- Bacterial Vaginosis

- Yeast Infection "Candida"

- Trichomoniasis vaginitis

- Human Papillomavirus (HPV)

- Genital Herpes

- Gonorrhea

- Chlamydia

- Vulvodynia

- Atrophic Vaginitis

CHAPTER TWO

VAGINAL ATROPHY

Atrophic vaginitis is a disorder that happens when your body generates less estrogen, generally after menopause. It leads to dryness, thinning, and inflammation of a woman's vaginal walls. Symptoms may include vaginal dryness, a burning feeling while peeing, minor blood after intercourse, and genital itching.

For many women, vaginal shrinkage not only makes intercourse unpleasant but also leads to severe urine symptoms. Because the illness produces both vaginal and urine symptoms, clinicians use the term "genitourinary syndrome of menopause (GSM)" to characterize vaginal atrophy and its concomitant symptoms.

Is Atrophic Vaginitis Contagious?

No, this is a condition women encounter owing to low amounts of estrogen. It cannot be transferred to a sexual partner, yet it may alter a woman's sexual experience. The incorporation of a sexual lubricant might relieve the pain associated with vaginal dryness.

SYMPTOMS

Genitourinary syndrome of menopause (GSM) signs and symptoms may include:

- Vaginal dryness
- Vaginal burning
- Vaginal discharge
- Genital itching
- Burning with urination
- Urgency with urinating
- Frequent urination
- Recurrent urinary tract infections
- Urinary incontinence

- Light bleeding after intercourse
- Discomfort with intercourse
- Decreased vaginal lubrication during sexual activity
- Shortening and tightness of the vaginal canal

When To Visit A Doctor

Many postmenopausal women suffer from GSM. But few seek treatment. Women may be ashamed to address their problems with their doctor and may resign themselves to live with these symptoms.

Make an appointment with your doctor if you have any unexplained vaginal spotting or bleeding, odd discharge, burning, or pain.

Also, schedule an appointment to visit your doctor if you suffer painful intercourse that's not eased by applying a vaginal moisturizer

CAUSES

- Normal vaginal lining vs. dry vaginal lining
- Vaginal drynessOpen pop-up dialog box
- Genitourinary syndrome of menopause is caused by a reduction in estrogen production. Less estrogen makes your vaginal tissues thinner, drier, less elastic, and more delicate.

A Reduction In Estrogen Levels May Occur:
- After menopause
- During the years coming up to menopause (perimenopause)
- After surgical excision of both ovaries (surgical menopause)
- During breast-feeding
- While using drugs that might influence estrogen levels, such as certain birth control pills
- After pelvic radiation treatment for cancer
- After treatment for cancer

- As a side effect of breast cancer hormonal

TREATMENT

GSM signs and symptoms may begin to annoy you during the years preceding menopause, or they may not become a problem until many years after menopause. Although the syndrome is frequent, not all menopausal women have GSM. Regular sexual activity, with or without a partner, may help you maintain healthy vaginal tissues.

RISK FACTORS

Certain variables may contribute to GSM, such as:

Smoking. Cigarette smoking affects your blood circulation and may limit the supply of blood and oxygen to the vagina and other adjacent locations. Smoking also lowers the impact of naturally produced estrogens in your body.

No vaginal births. Researchers have noticed that women who have never given birth vaginally are more prone to have GSM symptoms than those who have had vaginal births.

No sexual activity. Sexual activity, with or without a partner, stimulates blood flow and makes your vaginal tissues more elastic.

COMPLICATIONS

Genitourinary syndrome of menopause raises your chances of:

- Vaginal infections.

Changes in the acid balance of your vagina make vaginal infections more frequent.

- Urinary issues.

Urinary alterations related to GSM might lead to urinary issues. You can have increased frequency or urgency of urinating or burning with pee. Some women develop increased urinary tract infections or urine leaks (incontinence).

PREVENTION

Regular sexual activity, either with or without a partner, may help avoid the genitourinary syndrome of menopause. Sexual activity boosts blood flow to your vagina, which helps maintain vaginal tissues healthy.

CHAPTER THREE

CHLAMYDIA

Sexually active females younger than 25 years, as well as older women with risk factors such as having new or many sex partners, or a sex partner who has a sexually transmitted infection, require testing every year.

Sexually active people may obtain chlamydia, a prevalent, curable, sexually transmitted illness (STD). This information sheet addresses general questions concerning chlamydia.

WHAT IS CHLAMYDIA?

Chlamydia is a prevalent STD that may cause infection in both men and women. It may cause lasting harm to a woman's reproductive system. This might make it difficult or impossible to become pregnant later. Chlamydia may also produce a potentially dangerous ectopic pregnancy (pregnancy that develops outside the womb).

HOW IS CHLAMYDIA SPREAD?

You can catch chlamydia by having vaginal, anal, or oral intercourse with someone who has chlamydia. Also, you may still develop chlamydia even if your sex partner does not ejaculate (cum). A pregnant individual with chlamydia might spread the illness to their kid after birthing.

How Can I Lower My Chance Of Acquiring Chlamydia?

The only method to entirely prevent STDs is to not have vaginal, anal, or oral intercourse.

If you are sexually active, the following activities might minimize your chances of having chlamydia:

Being in a long-term mutually monogamous relationship with a partner who has been tested and does not have chlamydia; and Appropriately using condoms every time you have sex.

Am I At Risk For Chlamydia?

Sexually active persons may obtain chlamydia via vaginal, anal, or oral intercourse without a condom with a partner who has chlamydia.
Sexually active young individuals are at a greater risk of contracting chlamydia. This is related to behavioral and biological variables prevalent among young individuals. Gay and bisexual men are particularly in danger as chlamydia may spread via oral and anal intercourse.

If you are sexually active, have an honest and open chat with your healthcare physician. Ask them whether you should be tested for chlamydia or other STDs. Gay or bisexual males and pregnant individuals should also be tested for chlamydia. If you are a sexually active woman, you should be tested for chlamydia every year if you are: YOUNGER THAN 25 YEARS OLD.

25 years and older with risk factors, such as having new or many sex partners, or a sex partner who has a sexually transmitted virus.

I'm Pregnant. How Can Chlamydia Harm My Kid?

If you are pregnant and have chlamydia, you may pass the illness to your kid during delivery. This might trigger an eye infection or pneumonia in your infant. Having chlamydia may also make it more probable to birth your baby early.

If you are pregnant, you should obtain a test for chlamydia at your first prenatal appointment. Talk to your healthcare professional about receiving the necessary evaluation, testing, and treatment. Testing and treatment are the greatest strategies to avoid health concerns.

How Can I Tell If I Have Chlamydia?

Chlamydia frequently has no symptoms, yet it may create major health issues, even without symptoms. If symptoms arise, they may not present until several weeks after having intercourse with a partner who has chlamydia.

Even though chlamydia has no symptoms, it may harm a woman's reproductive system. Women with symptoms may notice

- An abnormal vaginal discharge
- A scorching feeling while peeing.

Symptoms in men may include

- A discharge from their penis;
- A scorching feeling while peeing; and
- Pain and swelling in one or both testicles (although this is less common).

Men and women may also have chlamydia in their rectum. This occurs either by having receptive anal intercourse or by transmission from another infected place (such as the vagina). While these diseases frequently create no symptoms, they may cause:

- Rectal pain;
- Discharge; and
- Bleeding.

See a healthcare physician if you detect any of these symptoms. You should also consult a physician if your spouse has an STD or signs of one.

SYMPTOMS MIGHT INCLUDE:

- An uncommon sore
- A stinky discharge
- Burning during peeing
- Bleeding between periods.

How Will My Healthcare Provider Know If I Have Chlamydia?

Laboratory testing can detect chlamydia. Your healthcare professional may ask you to submit a urine sample for testing, or they could use (or urge you to use) a cotton swab to acquire a vaginal sample.

Is There A Treatment For Chlamydia?

Yes, the appropriate medicine can cure chlamydia. You must take all of the medication your healthcare practitioner prescribes to treat your infection. Do not share drugs for chlamydia with anybody.

When used correctly it will stop the illness and possibly minimize your chances of experiencing difficulties later. Although treatment will eliminate the illness, it will not restore any chronic harm caused by the sickness.

Repeat infection with chlamydia is frequent. You should undergo testing again around three months following your therapy, even if your sex partner(s) receives treatment.

When Can I Have Sex Again After My Chlamydia Treatment?

You should not have sex again until you and your sex partner(s) finish therapy. If given a single dosage of medication, you should wait seven days after taking the drug before having intercourse. If given medication to take for seven days, wait until you complete all the doses before having sex.

If you've had chlamydia and taken treatment in the past, you may still acquire it again. This may happen if you have intercourse without a condom with a person who has chlamydia.

What Happens If I Don't Get Treated?

The early harm that chlamydia does sometimes goes unreported. However, chlamydia may lead to major health complications.

In women, untreated chlamydia may cause pelvic inflammatory disease (PID). Some of the complications of PID are:
- Formation of scar tissue that clogs fallopian tubes;
- Ectopic pregnancy (pregnancy outside the womb);
- Infertility (not being able to become pregnant); and
- Long-term pelvic/abdominal discomfort.

Men seldom experience health complications from chlamydia. The infection may produce fever and discomfort in the tubes connecting to the testicles. This may, in rare situations, lead to infertility.

Untreated chlamydia may also raise your risk of developing or donating HIV.

CHAPTER FOUR

YEAST INFECTION (VAGINAL)

Yeast infections are fungal infections that result in discharge, discomfort, and an exceedingly painful itching feeling on the vulva and vagina. Resuming a sexual activity after a time of abstinence may lead to yeast infections and some research points to oral sex is a cause as well.

Also termed vaginal candidiasis, vaginal yeast infection affects up to 3 out of 4 women at some point in their lives. Many women endure at least two episodes.

A vaginal yeast infection isn't considered a sexually transmitted infection. But, there's an elevated chance of vaginal yeast infection at the time of first regular sexual activity. There's also some indication that illnesses may be connected to mouth-to-genital contact (oral-genital sex).

Medications may successfully cure vaginal yeast infections. If you have recurring yeast infections — four or more within a year — you may require a lengthier treatment course and a maintenance plan.

SYMPTOMS

Yeast infection symptoms may vary from mild to severe, and include:

- Itching and discomfort in the vagina and vulva
- A scorching feeling, particularly during intercourse or during urinating
- Redness and swelling of the vulva
- Vaginal discomfort and tenderness
- Vaginal rash
- Thick, white, odor-free vaginal discharge with a cottage cheese look

- Watery vaginal discharge

COMPLICATED YEAST INFECTION:

You could have a complex yeast infection if:
- You experience severe signs and symptoms, such as widespread redness, swelling, and itching that leads to tears, splits, or sores
- You get four or more yeast infections in a year
- Your illness is caused by a less usual form of fungus
- You're pregnant
- You have uncontrolled diabetes
- Your immune system is impaired because of certain drugs or illnesses such as HIV infection

When To Visit A Doctor

Make an appointment with your doctor if:

- This is the first time you've encountered yeast infection symptoms
- You're not sure if you have a yeast infection
- Your symptoms aren't improved after treatment with over-the-counter antifungal vaginal creams or suppositories
- You experience additional symptoms

CAUSES

The fungus candida Albicans is responsible for most vaginal yeast infections.

Your vagina naturally contains a balanced mix of yeast, including candida, and bacteria. Certain bacteria (lactobacillus) work to inhibit the overgrowth of yeast.

But that equilibrium may be upset. An overgrowth of candida or penetration of the fungus into deeper vaginal cell layers produces the signs and symptoms of a yeast infection.

Overgrowth Of Yeast May Originate From:

- Antibiotic usage, which produces an imbalance in natural vaginal flora
- Pregnancy
- Uncontrolled diabetes
- A weakened immune system
- Taking oral contraception or hormone treatment that enhances estrogen levels
- Candida albicans is the most prevalent form of fungus that cause yeast infections. Yeast infections caused by other forms of candida fungus may be more difficult to cure and often require more-aggressive medications.

RISK FACTORS

Factors that enhance your chance of having a yeast infection include:

Antibiotic Usage:
Yeast infections are prevalent in women who take antibiotics. Broad-spectrum antibiotics, which kill a variety of germs, also destroy good bacteria in your vagina, leading to the overgrowth of yeast.

Increased Estrogen Levels.
Yeast infections are more frequent in women with greater estrogen levels — such as pregnant women or women using high-dose estrogen birth control pills or estrogen

Hormone Treatment.
Uncontrolled diabetes. Women with poorly managed blood sugar are at increased risk of yeast infections than women with well-controlled blood sugar.

Impaired Immune System.
Women with decreased immunity — such as from corticosteroid medication or HIV

infection — are more prone to yeast infections.

PREVENTION

To lower your risk of vaginal yeast infections, wear underwear that has a cotton crotch and doesn't fit too tightly.

It could also assist to avoid:

Tight-fitting pantyhose
Douching, which destroys part of the usual bacteria in the vagina that protect you against infection
Scented feminine items, including bubble baths, pads, and tampons
Hot pools and really hot baths
Unnecessary antibiotic usages, such as for colds or other viral diseases
Staying in wet garments, such as swimwear and gym apparel, for lengthy periods but

CHAPTER FIVE

TRICHOMONIASIS

Trichomoniasis is a common sexually transmitted illness caused by a parasite. Symptoms vary from person to person and may also include discomfort while peeing and a change in discharge and vaginal odor, genital itching, and painful urination.

Men who have trichomoniasis often have no symptoms. Pregnant mothers who have trichomoniasis can be at increased risk of delivering their newborns prematurely.

Is Trichomoniasis Contagious?

Yes, trichomoniasis is a sexually transmitted illness. The only certain approach to avoiding the contraction of any STD is abstinence. However, frequent check-ups and conversations with your partner together with the use of condoms help to lower your risks of acquiring trichomoniasis.

TREATMENT FOR TRICHOMONIASIS

is taking an antibiotic — either metronidazole (Flagyl), tinidazole (Tindamax) or secnidazole (Solosec). To avoid becoming infected again, all sexual partners should be treated at the same time. You may lower your chance of infection by wearing condoms appropriately every time you have sex.

SYMPTOMS

Trichomoniasis symptoms may be hard to detect and may come and go, so most individuals don't realize they have it. If you do see indications of trich, get tested soon away.

Often trichomoniasis has no symptoms.
About 7 out of 10 patients with trich exhibit no indications of the illness at all. When the infection is in a penis, it's quite uncommon to create symptoms. Sometimes the symptoms of trich are so subtle that you don't even notice them, or you assume it's a separate illness (like a yeast infection or a UTI). So the only way to find out for sure whether you have it is to be tested.

SYMPTOMS OF TRICHOMONIASIS

If you do acquire symptoms of trichomoniasis, they generally show up from 3 days to a month after you get the illness.

Trichomoniasis may induce symptoms in persons of either gender. But trich is more likely to induce vaginitis. Symptoms of vaginitis induced by trich include:

Green, yellow, gray, foamy, and/or bad-smelling vaginal discharge

Blood in your vaginal discharge
- Itching and discomfort in and around your vagina
- Swelling around your genitals
- Pain during sex

Other symptoms of trich include discomfort and burning when you urinate, the need to pee a lot, discharge from your urethra, and itching and irritation within your penis.

The indicators of trich might be scarcely detectable, or highly unpleasant and bothersome. It's usual for the symptoms to come and go, but it doesn't indicate the infection went gone. The only option to get rid of trichomoniasis is to be treated with drugs.

If you or your sexual partner develops any of these symptoms, consult a nurse, doctor, or your local Planned Parenthood Health Center. You may transfer trich to other people whether or not you have symptoms, so it's crucial to be tested if you suspect you may be sick.

CAUSES

Trichomoniasis is caused by a one-celled protozoan, a kind of microscopic parasite called Trichomonas vaginitis. The parasite spreads between humans via genital contact, including vaginal, oral, or anal intercourse. The infection may be spread between males and women, women, and occasionally men.

The parasite attacks the lower genital tract. In women, this comprises the outside section of the genitals (vulva), vagina, the entrance of the uterus (cervix), and urine opening (urethra). In males, the parasite affects the interior of the penis (urethra).

The time between exposure to the parasite and infection (incubation period) is uncertain. But it's estimated to span from four to 28 days. Even without symptoms, you or your partner may still carry the illness.

RISK FACTORS

Risk factors for obtaining trichomoniasis include having:

- Multiple sexual partners
- A history of various sexually transmitted illnesses (STIs)
- A prior bout of trichomoniasis
- Sex without a condom

COMPLICATIONS

Pregnant women who have trichomoniasis might:

- Deliver too early (prematurely)
- Have a kid with a low birth weight

- Give the infection to the infant when the baby travels through the birth canal
- Having trichomoniasis produces inflammation in the vaginal region that may make it easier for other STIs to enter the body or to spread to others.
- Trichomoniasis also seems to make it easier to get infected with the human immunodeficiency virus (HIV), the virus that causes acquired immunodeficiency syndrome (AIDS).
- Trichomoniasis is related to an increased risk of cervical or prostate cancer.
- Untreated, trichomoniasis infection may linger for months to years.

PREVENTION

As with other sexually transmitted illnesses, the only approach to avoid trichomoniasis is to not have sex. To minimize your risk, wear internal or external condoms appropriately every time you have sex.

CHAPTER SIX

GENITAL HERPES

What Is Genital Herpes?

Genital herpes is a sexually transmitted infection (STI). It creates herpetic sores, which are painful blisters (fluid-filled lumps) that may burst apart and spill fluid.

CAUSES OF GENITAL HERPES

Genital herpes is caused by two viruses:

- HSV-1. This variety generally causes cold sores, but it may also cause genital herpes.

- HSV-2. This variety commonly causes genital herpes, although it may also cause cold sores.

The viruses enter the body via skin abrasions or mucous membranes. Mucous membranes are the thin layers of tissue that line the openings of your body. They may be discovered in your nose, mouth, and genitals.

Once the viruses are inside the body, they integrate themselves into the cells. Viruses tend to reproduce or adapt to their settings extremely quickly, which makes treating them challenging.

HSV-1 or HSV-2 may be discovered in body fluids, including:

- Saliva
- Semen
- Vaginal secretions

The emergence of blisters is known as an outbreak. On average, a first outbreak would show 4 days, after getting the virus, according to the Centers for Disease Control and Prevention (CDC). However, it might take as little as 2 days, or as much as 12 days or more, to show.

General Symptoms For Persons With A Penis Include Blisters On The:
- Penis
- Scrotum
- Buttocks(near or around the anus)

General Symptoms For Persons With A Vagina Include Blisters Around The:
- Vagina
- Anus
- Buttocks

Is Herpes Contagious?

Yes, genital herpes is a prevalent sexually transmitted illness. Even when a person does not display any symptoms, the STD is still infectious.

General Symptoms For Anybody Include The Following:

- Blisters may occur in the mouth and on the lips, face, and anyplace else that comes into touch with regions of infection.
- The region that has developed the illness frequently begins to itch, or tingle, before blisters emerge.
- The blisters may become ulcerated (open sores) and exude fluid.
- A crust may grow over the sores within a week of the onset.
- The lymph glands may become enlarged. Lymph glands combat infection and inflammation in the body.
- The viral infection may induce headaches, body pains, and fever.

General symptoms for a newborn born with herpes (contracted HSV during a vaginal birth) may include sores on the face, torso, and genitals.

Babies who are born with genital herpes may develop extremely serious problems and experience:

- Blindness
- Brain Damage
- Death

It's extremely crucial to inform a doctor if there's a current genital herpes diagnosis or if HSV is caught while pregnant so that they will take efforts to prevent the virus from being spread to an unborn baby during delivery. If there are herpes blisters along the birth canal, the healthcare team may elect to deliver the baby through cesarean rather than a typical vaginal delivery.

ORAL HERPES AND COLD SORES

Cold sores are a sign of oral herpes (HSV-1). Cold sores are blister-like lesions that form around the mouth or lips. They may also arise on other parts of the face. They often last for 2 weeks or longer. Because there's no treatment for herpes, cold sores might come back.

How Frequent Is Genital Herpes?

Genital herpes is extremely frequent, although genital herpes is primarily caused by HSV-2, the illness may also be caused by HSV-1.

When To Visit A Doctor For Genital Herpes

If there are no signs of genital herpes, the CDC does not suggest being tested for herpes.

However, if there are signs of genital herpes, it's crucial to contact a doctor. They can provide a diagnosis and discuss care solutions for the infection.

Additionally, if there's a likelihood of having been exposed to HSV, or if there's a wish to obtain a comprehensive STI check and testing, it's encouraged to book an appointment with a doctor.

If an in-person visit is not feasible, an at-home test kit is another option to explore. However, it's crucial to remember that an in-person test done by a doctor may be more accurate.

DIAGNOSING GENITAL HERPES

A doctor may often identify a herpes transmission by a visual examination of the herpes lesions. Although testing is not always essential, a doctor may confirm their diagnosis using laboratory tests.

A blood test may identify HSV before an epidemic begins. However, if there has not been contacting with the virus and no symptoms are being presented, it's not necessarily required to get examined for HSV-1 or HSV-2.

Ordering a home test kit for herpes might be an option to investigate.

Can Genital Herpes Be Treated?

Treatment may minimize outbreaks, but it cannot cure herpes simplex viruses.

MEDICATIONS

Antiviral medications may help speed up the healing period for sores and minimize discomfort. Medications may be given at the earliest indications of an outbreak (tingling, and other symptoms) to help minimize the symptoms.

If there have been outbreaks, a doctor may also prescribe drugs to make it less likely that new outbreaks would develop.

HOME CARE

Use mild cleansers while bathing or showering in warm water. Keep the afflicted location clean and dry. Wear loose cotton garments to keep the region comfortable.

How Genital Herpes Is Spread

HSV is spread by sexual interaction, which might include:
- Vaginal sex
- Anal sex
- Any additional behaviors that entail touch between genitals

It's possible to develop an HSV infection via oral sex. Oral herpes may spread to the vaginal and anal regions and vice versa.

Although HSV is generally spread via skin-to-skin contact, the virus may also be detected in semen, saliva, and vaginal fluids.

RISK FACTORS for getting genital herpes
The chance of developing HSV rises in several settings, including:

- Having vaginal, oral, or anal intercourse with someone who has genital herpes
- Without using condoms or other barrier techniques while having sex
- Having a diminished capacity to fend off infection (compromised immune system), owing to another STI or sickness

PREVENTING GENITAL HERPES

If a person is sexually active, they may minimize their chance of developing HSV by:
- Using barrier devices, like condoms, every time they have sex.
- Refraining from intercourse with someone who is exhibiting herpes signs. However, it's vital to realize that HSV may be given to another person even when symptoms are not evident.
- Talking with sexual partners about their STI status.

What to do after testing positive for genital herpes

If a person tests positive for genital herpes, it's suggested that they consult with a doctor. Although there's no cure for herpes, it may be managed using antiviral treatment.

Antiviral medicine may help minimize the intensity of repeated outbreaks (both cold sores and genital warts).

Frequent, severe recurring breakouts could be an indication of a damaged immune system. If outbreaks are happening regularly, a doctor could explore if there's an underlying problem impacting the immune system.

Having sex is OK if there's a genital herpes diagnosis, but it's preferable to avoid sex if there's a herpes outbreak. To limit the possibility of spreading HSV to a partner, utilize barrier techniques such as condoms and dental dams during any sexual activity.

What Happens If Genital Herpes Stays Untreated?

Genital herpes may not usually need treatment. However, genital warts may be uncomfortable. Antiviral therapy may lower the symptoms and intensity of outbreaks.
In rare circumstances, herpes might create difficulties. Generally, however, it does not become worse with time.

What Should I Know If I Am Pregnant And I Have Genital Herpes?

It's reasonable to be anxious about the health of your kid when you have any form of STI. HSV may be passed to your kid if you have an aggressive outbreak during vaginal birth.

It's crucial to notify your doctor that you have genital herpes as soon as you discover you're pregnant.

Your doctor will describe what to anticipate before, during, and after you deliver your baby. They may prescribe pregnancy-safe medicines to ensure a healthy birth. They may also elect to deliver their baby by cesarean.

Long-term prospects for genital herpes
Practicing safer sex and using condoms or another barrier device every time you have sexual contact with someone is vital. It will help avoid developing and spreading HSV and other STIs.

There's currently no treatment for genital herpes, although researchers are working on producing a cure or vaccine.
However, the illness may be treated with medicine.

The illness sits latent inside the body until something sparks an epidemic. Outbreaks might arise owing to being worried, unwell, or fatigued.

A doctor can assist design a treatment plan to control breakouts.

You might asked!

What Does A Herpes Sore Look Like?

Herpes sores first seem like little pus-filled lumps, similar to pimples or blisters. These lesions might burst open and exude fluids, which produces a crust. It might seem like one sore on its own, or there can be a cluster of sores.

Herpes sores may appear on the skin surrounding the mouth (cold sores) or around the genitals or anus.

What Are The Earliest Indications of Genital Herpes In A Woman?

One of the earliest indicators of genital herpes in women is itchy or tingling skin, which gives a lead to herpes ulcers. This might arise near the vagina or anus.

Women could also have flu-like symptoms, including fever and exhaustion. Headaches, bodily pains, and lymph node swelling may also develop due to an HSV infection.

Remember, however, that it's possible to have an HSV-2 infection without presenting any symptoms.

How Did Genital Herpes Initially Appear?

Genital herpes lesions initially form a few days after exposure. According to the CDC, the initial outbreak generally emerges 4 days, after getting the virus (although it can take as little as 2 days, or as much as 12 days or more).

The sores will initially seem like tiny, fluid-filled pimples or blisters. After a few days, the fluid pours out of the pimples. The sores crust up before healing.

Is Genital Herpes Infectious For Life?

A person is more likely to spread HSV while they're experiencing an outbreak — that is when the herpes sores initially emerge until they're entirely healed. However, even in latent times (between outbreaks), it is possible to transfer HSV to a partner.

To limit the possibility of spreading HSV during sexual contact, employ a barrier technique like condoms and dental dams during every sexual activity.

CHAPTER SEVEN

GONORRHEA

Gonorrhea is an infection caused by a sexually transmitted bacteria that affects both men and females. Gonorrhea most typically affects the urethra, rectum, or throat. In females, gonorrhea may also infect the cervix.

Gonorrhea is most usually transferred through vaginal, oral, or anal intercourse. But kids of sick moms may be infected during delivery. In newborns, gonorrhea most usually affects the eyes.

Is Gonorrhea Contagious?

Yes, gonorrhea is a sexually transmitted illness. When acquired, this STD is treated with antibiotics. So long as treatment is taken as recommended, gonorrhea may be healed. However, if the STD has caused chronic harm, the therapy does not cure any of those consequences.

Abstaining from sex, wearing a condom if you have sex, and being in a mutually monogamous relationship are the greatest strategies to avoid sexually transmitted illnesses.

SYMPTOMS

Male reproductive system

The male reproductive system opens pop-up dialog box locations of female reproductive organs

Female reproductive system open pop-up dialog box

In many situations, gonorrhea infection generates no symptoms. Symptoms, however, may impact numerous areas in your body but are typically present in the genital system.

Gonorrhea affecting the vaginal tract

Signs and symptoms of gonorrhea infection in men include:

- Painful urination
- Pus-like discharge from the tip of the penis
- Pain or swelling in one testicle

Signs and symptoms of gonorrhea infection in women include:

- Increased vaginal discharge
- Painful urination
- Vaginal bleeding between periods, such as after vaginal intercourse
- Abdominal or pelvic pain

Gonorrhea may also affect various sections of the body such as:

RECTUM

Signs and symptoms include anal irritation, pus-like discharge from the rectum, specks of bright red blood on toilet paper, and needing to strain during bowel movements.

EYES
Gonorrhea that affects your eyes may cause eye discomfort, sensitivity to light, and pus-like discharge from one or both eyes.

THROAT
Signs and symptoms of a throat infection could include a painful throat and enlarged lymph nodes in the neck.

JOINTS
If one or more joints get infected by bacteria (septic arthritis), the afflicted joints could be warm, red, swollen, and exceedingly painful, particularly during movement.

WHEN TO VISIT YOUR DOCTOR

Make an appointment with your doctor if you detect any concerning signs or symptoms, such as a burning feeling when you pee or a pus-like discharge from your penis, vagina, or rectum.

Also, arrange an appointment with your doctor if your spouse has been diagnosed with gonorrhea. You may not have signs or symptoms that encourage you to seek medical assistance. But without therapy, you may reinfect your partner even after he or she has been treated for gonorrhea.

CAUSES

Gonorrhea is caused by the bacteria Neisseria gonorrhoeae. Gonorrhea germs are most typically spread from one person to another via sexual contact, including oral, anal, or vaginal intercourse.

RISK FACTORS

Sexually active women younger than 25 and males who have intercourse with men are at higher risk of contracting gonorrhea.

Other variables that might raise your risk include:
- Having a new sex partner
- Having a sex partner who has other partners
- Having more than one sex partner
- Having experienced gonorrhea or another sexually transmitted illness

COMPLICATIONS

Untreated gonorrhea may lead to serious consequences, such as:

Infertility In Women.
Gonorrhea may extend into the uterus and fallopian tubes, producing pelvic inflammatory disease (PID). PID may result in scarring of the tubes, a higher risk of

pregnancy difficulties, and infertility. PID needs urgent

Infertility In Males.
Gonorrhea may cause a tiny, coiled tube in the posterior section of the testicles where the sperm ducts are situated (epididymis) to become inflamed (epididymitis). Untreated epididymitis may lead to infertility.

Infection That Spreads To The Joints And Other Regions Of Your Body.
The bacteria that cause gonorrhea may move via the circulation and infect other areas of your body, including your joints. Fever, rash, skin lesions, joint discomfort, edema, and stiffness are potential effects.

Increased Risk Of Hiv/aids.
Having gonorrhea makes you more vulnerable to infection with the human immunodeficiency virus (HIV), the virus that leads to AIDS. People who have both

gonorrhea and HIV can spread both infections more easily to their partners.

COMPLICATIONS IN INFANTS.

Babies who get gonorrhea from their mothers after birth might have blindness, lesions on the scalp, and infections.

PREVENTION

- Use a condom if you have sex.

Abstaining from sex is the surest approach to avoid gonorrhea. But if you want to have sex, wear a condom during any sort of sexual contact, including anal sex, oral sex, or vaginal intercourse.

- Limit your amount of sex partners.

Being in a monogamous relationship in which neither partner has sex with anybody else may minimize your risk.

- Be sure you and your partner get checked for sexually transmitted illnesses.

Before you have sex, get tested and communicate your findings with each other.

- Don't have sex with someone who looks to have a sexually transmitted infection.

- If your partner has signs or symptoms of a sexually transmitted illness, such as burning during urination or a genital rash or soreness, don't have intercourse with that individual.

- Consider frequent gonorrhea screening.

Annual screening is advised for sexually active women younger than 25 and older women at greater risk of infection. This covers women who have a new sex partner, more than one sex partner, a sex partner with other partners, or a sex partner who has a sexually transmitted virus.

- Regular screening is also suggested for males who have sex with men, as well as their partners.

- To prevent acquiring gonorrhea again, refrain from sex until after you and your sex partner have finished therapy and after the symptoms are gone.

CHAPTER EIGHT

BACTERIAL VAGINOSIS

Bacterial Vaginosis (BV) develops when bacteria grow up in the vagina. Since maintaining balance is crucial for the vagina, BV results in atypical discharge, itching or soreness in the vagina, and a distinct fishy smell that is particularly noticeable during sexual intercourse.

Although the reason is not fully known by experts, it does seem sexually active women are more likely to have BV.

<u>Is Bacterial Vaginosis Contagious?</u>

While you can't obtain BV from surfaces like toilet seats, it does seem that sex and douching have a part in the disturbance of vaginal balance, and having BV does put women at risk for developing other sexually transmitted diseases (STDs).

Women in their reproductive years are more prone to have bacterial vaginosis, although it may afflict women of any age. The reason isn't known, although certain practices, such as unprotected intercourse or regular douching, enhance your risk.

SYMPTOMS

Bacterial vaginosis signs and symptoms may include:
- Thin, gray, white, or green vaginal discharge
- Foul-smelling "fishy" vaginal odor
- Vaginal itching
- Burning during urinating

Many women with bacterial vaginosis have no indications or symptoms.

When To Visit A Doctor

Make an appointment to visit your doctor if:
- You experience vaginal discharge that's new and linked with an odor or temperature. Your doctor can assist

diagnose the reason and identify indications and symptoms.

- You've experienced vaginal infections previously, but the color and substance of your discharge look different this time.

- You have several sex partners or a recent new relationship. Sometimes, the signs and symptoms of a sexually transmitted illness are identical to those of bacterial vaginosis.

- You attempt self-treatment for yeast infection using an over-the-counter remedy and your symptoms linger.

CAUSES

Bacterial vaginosis develops from the overgrowth of one of the numerous bacteria normally occurring in your vagina. Usually, "healthy" bacteria (lactobacilli) outweigh "bad" bacteria (anaerobes). But if there are too many anaerobic bacteria, they disturb the normal balance of microorganisms in your vagina and cause bacterial vaginosis.

RISK FACTORS

Risk factors for bacterial vaginosis include:
- Having several sex partners or a new sex partner.

Doctors don't completely understand the relationship between sexual activity and bacterial vaginosis, although the illness occurs more commonly in women who have several sex partners or a new sex partner. Bacterial vaginosis also occurs more commonly in women who have intercourse with women.

- Douching.

The technique of washing out your vagina with water or a cleaning chemical (douching) disrupts the natural equilibrium of your vagina. This may lead to an excess of anaerobic bacteria, and cause bacterial vaginosis. Since the vagina is self-cleaning, douching isn't essential.

- Natural deficiency of lactobacilli bacteria.

If your natural vaginal environment doesn't create enough of the healthy lactobacilli bacteria, you're more likely to get bacterial vaginosis.

COMPLICATIONS

Bacterial vaginosis doesn't often create difficulties. Sometimes, having bacterial vaginosis may lead to:

- Preterm birth.

In pregnant women, bacterial vaginosis is connected to early births and low birth weight newborns.

- Sexually transmitted infections.

Having bacterial vaginosis renders women more vulnerable to sexually transmitted illnesses, such as HIV, herpes simplex virus, chlamydia, or gonorrhea. If you have HIV, bacterial vaginosis raises the likelihood that you'll transfer the infection to your partner.

- Infection risk following gynecologic surgery.

Having bacterial vaginosis may raise the chance of acquiring a post-surgical infection following operations such as hysterectomy or dilatation and curettage (D&C).

- Pelvic inflammatory illness (PID).

Bacterial vaginosis may occasionally develop PID, an infection of the uterus and the fallopian tubes that can raise the risk of infertility.

PREVENTION

- Minimize vaginal irritation.

Use moderate, nondeodorant soaps and unscented tampons or pads.

- Don't douche.

Your vagina doesn't need cleaning other than routine bathing. Frequent douching alters the vaginal balance and may raise your risk of vaginal infection. Douching won't clean up a vaginal infection.

- Avoid a sexually transmitted illness.

Use a male latex condom, restrict your number of sex partners or refrain from intercourse to lessen your chance of a sexually transmitted infection.

CONCLUSION

While it might be worrisome to face the risk of acquiring a vaginal illness, you should always prioritize your feminine care. If you have any symptoms of the vaginal disorders described above consult your doctor.

<u>What Can I Anticipate If I Have Vaginitis?</u>

Vaginitis is painful, but understanding the reason and the correct therapy might provide you relief. If chemical irritants are causing your vaginitis, you may improve your symptoms by avoiding the bothersome lotion, detergent, spray, etc. Bacterial and antifungal drugs may take up to two weeks to clear your illness. Antiviral drugs for viral vaginitis can't cure the infection, but they may help your symptoms to go away quicker. Getting the appropriate diagnosis and addressing the causes of your vaginitis is crucial when it comes to curing your symptoms.

Follow your healthcare provider's instructions, as well as the instructions that come with any medicine you're taking for vaginitis. Don't stop taking the drug when your symptoms go gone. Speak to your healthcare practitioner about any questions you have regarding your treatment or follow-up.

What Questions Should I Ask My Doctor?

Good questions to ask include:

- Should I refrain from sex during treatment?
- Should my sexual partner(s) be treated at the same time?
- How will the treatment for this vaginitis interact with my other medications?
- Should I continue the vaginal cream or suppositories throughout my period?

- Do I need to be re-examined and if so, when?

Don't be ashamed to speak to your physician about symptoms you're having that could be vaginitis. It's a common ailment that's manageable – if you find out what's causing your symptoms. The sooner you and your healthcare practitioner determine what's causing your pain, the sooner you may obtain the therapy required to offer you relief.